Helping Hands for Dental Hygienists

101 Timeless Treasures for a Successful Career

Linda M. Harvey, RDH

HORIZON CONSULTING GROUP, INC.

Jacksonville, Florida

Published by Horizon Consulting Group, Inc.
P.O. Box 7238
Jacksonvile, FL 32238

Publisher's Cataloging-in-Publication Data
Harvey, Linda M.
Helping hands for dental hygienists / Linda M. Harvey. —
Jacksonville, FL: Horizon Consulting Group, Inc., 2000.
p. cm.

ISBN 0-9678758-0-3
1. Dental hygiene—Vocational guidance.
2. Dental hygienists. I. Title.
RK60 .H37 2000 00-100804
617.6/01 DC—21 CIP

PROJECT COORDINATION BY JENKINS GROUP, INC.

03 02 01 00 ✦ 5 4 3 2 1

Printed in the United States of America

To my family and in loving memory of my father,
I cherish your unconditional love and encouragement
in all my endeavors.

Contents

Acknowledgements

The words of wisdom in this book represent decades of dental hygiene experience. Dental hygienists across the nation extended their hands and hearts to contribute to this book. It is truly a privilege and a blessing to know so many talented, giving, dedicated individuals.

To all the wonderful hygienists who so enthusiastically gave their time and talents, I express my heartfelt gratitude.

To my special friends in the Northeast Florida Component, I thank you for your continual support. You are my inspiration.

Introduction

Registered Dental Hygienists are very special and unique individuals. Their many talents far exceed the instrumentation skills that they all struggled with in school. The role of a hygienist represents a combination of clinician, teacher, educator, comforter and counselor. The multitude of these talents is displayed throughout the chapters of this book in their timeless words of wisdom.

Many of the contributors have completed advanced degrees and some have taken on challenges beyond clinical practice. Nonetheless, they all share a common beginning as a Registered Dental Hygienist. They also share a similar journey marked by changes, growth and opportunities throughout the years. As a result, these individuals eagerly offer advice so that others may benefit. Regardless of where you are on your professional journey, you will find their treasures invaluable for a successful career.

Chapter One

Why We Do What We Do

I am blessed because I chose a profession that over the years became more than a job, it became a passion. That passion came from the people I met and continue to meet every day. Everyone in life should have a passion about something and if you are lucky enough to find your passion in your work, then I believe your life is truly good.

Fran Pangakis, RDH
1971

I believe a person can have all the technical skills of being a dental hygienist but it takes heart (i.e., being a compassionate, caring person) to fully care for a patient. Heart is something you cannot teach. It comes naturally from within.

Patricia Baughman, RDH, RN
1990

Be PROUD that you are a dental hygienist. I have seen thousands of patients over the past 30 years and every day while practicing there was something that occurred to me. It may have been the first, last, or any of the patients in between, but it happened every day. At some point while I was working with the patient, I would realize precisely what I was doing with the instruments. You see, YOU are taking YOUR two hands and making those instruments do exactly what they were designed to do. YOU are performing a precise art and it is like a ballet. There is a real sense of pride, which is defined as, "That which compels a person to do his or her best work especially when no one is looking."

Robert W. Ankrom, RDH, BS
1969

Be creative in defining how you'll be a dental hygienist. Too often, we can fall into a rut. Clinical practice may be just what you're looking for at one time in your life. At some other time, teaching or working in the dental industry may seem more appealing. I've been fortunate to have had many experiences as a dental hygienist. Not one of them was actually a position waiting to be filled. Know what you do well and what you enjoy. You'll be suited to fill that position! Dental hygiene practice isn't limited to seeing patients in a clinical setting. The skills and knowledge that you have enable you to choose a job in a variety of settings. You don't stop being a dental hygienist, you just may do it in a slightly different way!

Judy O'Brien, RDH, BA
1978

Dental hygiene has been the foundation of my success. I use almost every skill that I used as a clinical hygienist now as a nonclinical hygienist. One of the most important skills is professionalism. The projection of professionalism will serve as a constant forward movement to our profession. May you look to preserve traditions of excellence even as you achieve success.

Sherry Wilson Altman, BSDH
1983

I have been through so many different avenues trying to decide on the right career. Once I found hygiene, I knew it was for me. Dental hygiene is a profession that provides a tremendous amount of flexibility, which enables you to balance family and work. Two aspects that I really love about the profession are patient education and professional camaraderie. I find it very satisfying and rewarding to teach patients things about their oral health that they either didn't know or hadn't been taught before. I am also impressed by the many close friendships that hygienists enjoy with their colleagues.

Season H. Plato, RDH
2000

Remain truly dedicated to our profession of dental hygiene and never lose sight of those who supported you through thick and thin ... your family and friends.

Stacee J. White, RDH
1999

Be compassionate, caring and really listen to your patients. Observe everything about them, not just their oral health.

Susan Follmer, RDH
1966

View your patient as a whole person not just as 'teeth.' Develop interpersonal skills that build rapport and trust. Your patients will find their visits more pleasant and you will find your career more fulfilling.

Ramona Jones, RDH
1983

I have found success when working with clients if I try to give them something they didn't expect. I use a smile, a joke, a positive comment, or somehow give them hope that their condition isn't as bad as they first thought.

Olivia Willis, RDH
1998

Many people do not enjoy or are nervous about going to the dentist. I try to put the patient at ease by giving them a sincere compliment when they sit in the chair. My hope is to make them feel that I really do care about them and their oral health.

Betty Zumpano, RDH
1973

Remember that all of those teeth you are working so intimately with are attached to a live person with thoughts and feelings. Treat both of them (teeth and patient) with respect and you should have excellent results.

Janie A. Hill, RDH, MHS
1980

Take off your professional blinders and don't judge your patient based on appearance. If you prejudge what you think someone can afford, it will limit your treatment recommendations. A patient may just be interested in hearing all the treatment options. In the end, treat every patient with utmost respect.

Angie Patel, RDH, BS
1991

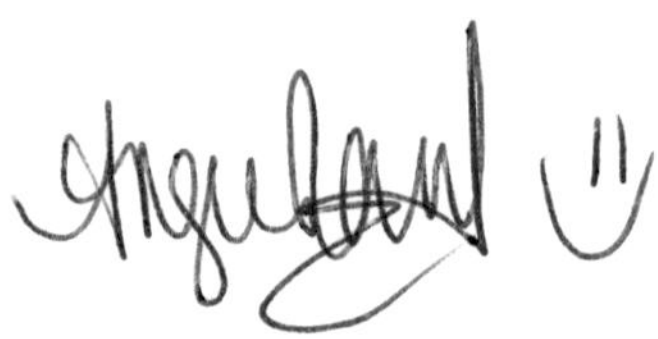

I have established a very close clientele of patients by having worked in one office since I graduated 13½ years ago. This becomes a big asset for you and your practice because you can follow patients' progress in their preventive care. Your patients become very comfortable with you and you with them. It's very rewarding to take care of your patients' dental needs and to help them understand the importance of good oral health.

Patty Dehner, RDH
1986

I love working with kids! Seeing them scared when they come in and happy when they leave is a very rewarding feeling. I accomplish this by making their visit fun and relating everything on their level. When children are happy patients, they grow into adults who love going to the dentist.

Renee Mackoul Klein, RDH
1962

When pediatric patients come in without smiles on their faces, I ask them if they "dropped" their smile on the ground. When they look at me, puzzled, I pretend to struggle while "picking up" their smile off the floor. They love this and it always brings their smile back.

Kaye Anne Sabaka, RDH
1997

The profession of dental hygiene will continuously be challenging whether working on a difficult patient or learning the ropes of a new office. If you are not happy with your work then you will not be successful. Positive thoughts and a smile will get you a long way. Your happiness is the most important and it isn't always derived from money.

Betty Dalton, RDH, BS
1987

I have experienced a most extraordinary, life-touching event that reminds me how special it is to be in this profession. For the past two years, I have been taking care of a former hygienist who has multiple sclerosis. When we first met, she could transfer herself from the wheelchair to the dental chair. I now attend to her oral health needs from her bed in the nursing home.

On one hand, it can be frustrating not being able to find help for certain patients within the system. On the other hand, I now know that anything is possible if we continually search for opportunities to make it happen.

Joann Grabowski, RDH
1970

Chapter Two

Shine Through Professionalism

A successful hygienist is one who:

- listens—there is always something to learn. The more you can learn about the total practice, the more valuable you are;

- tracks his or her production. Becoming business savvy is essential in today's practice. Understand the value you create in a practice;

- grows professionally by taking clinical and nonclinical courses. Improving communication, negotiation, and people skills is almost important as your clinical skills. Invest in your professional value.

Becky Heilman, RDH
1973

Successful people are successful
because they never gave up trying.

Jackie Burt McDonough, RDH
1979

Don't always take yourself and your work so seriously. Remember our co-workers are just as important as we are to the smooth running of the dental office. Try to find a little humor in the most stressful situations. Humor tends to lift a burden that wasn't there anyway. You'll be surprised to find out how much less stressful your day will be when you look for the lemonade when faced with the lemons.

Katherine A. Woods, RDH, MPH
1971

This profession has allowed me to touch people's lives far beyond the basics I learned in hygiene school. Through the years I have listened to people's problems, heard about their joyous moments, held their hands during the hard times, and most of all have had the privilege of calling many of them friends. I often say, "If I won the lottery tomorrow, I would still continue to practice, however I would only see the people I wanted to." And that would keep me working full-time!

Fran Pangakis, RDH
1971

Scale with a smile and treat your patients/clients as if they were loved ones.

Pamela S. Ridilla, RDH, BA
1980

Have you ever heard ... patients do not care what you know, only how much you care? Focus completely on them and pamper them as if you were in the chair. The little things count, such as lubricant on their lips, sunglasses for their eyes, topical anesthetic, rest breaks, being aware of their comfort zone, learning to read their body language, and being their informational source.

Being a professional registered dental hygienist is about TRUST. Trust is earned through credibility and personally caring.

Selene M. Beckworth, RDH, MEd
1975

A kind word and friendly smile can go a long way during your workday. Your patients want to feel good about themselves and you have the ability to change their attitude just by showing them you care.

Elizabeth Ellison, RDH
1989

In my station, I have a poem titled "Attitude." It is in clear view for my patients to see. It stresses that events in life are 10% and how we choose to react to them is 90%. This statement has started many a positive conversation. Not only do I feel we can improve the quality of our patients' oral health but when the occasion arises, we can influence their overall health as well.

Robin Gentry, RDH
1999

Go into an office with an open mind and be prepared to continue learning new things. You'll feel you learned it all in dental hygiene school. However, you will find that your skills and chairside manner will still be developing.

Jaymie Shipley, RDH
1999

Idle chatter is a deadly sin for the dental hygienist. Be friendly, interested, and genuine ... then "wow" them with what you know about new products, customized homecare coaching, or technology. Small talk is good for building rapport but use the patient's time wisely. They are paying for your hands and your knowledge. Know your stuff and show it off. Shine as the health care professional you are.

Jill C. Obrochta, RDH, BS
1984

Dental hygienists are highly skilled and educated in preventive oral health. Be sure each patient knows that you are the person to ask for information about how his or her oral health is affected by home care, diet, heredity, or medical intervention. Continually update your knowledge so that you will have the answers.

Howard M. Notgarnie, RDH, BA
1992

Learning something you did not know before is the best cure for burnout. It will renew your enthusiasm for your chosen profession. Man only sees what man knows ... the rest is hidden in plain view.

Victoria Barnett, RDH
1981

You worked very hard to achieve your status. You do not have a *job*, you have a *profession*. Give your patients, employer, and staff respect daily and expect no less from them in return.

Jolie Davis, RDH
1991

Treat every patient as you would want to be treated.

Gina Damico, RDH, MEd
1986

The biggest key to having a good day is being prepared. I never leave at night without preparing for the next day. I check the schedule, review charts, and have the appropriate instrument setups ready. This helps me to feel less pressured and be fully focused on my patients.

Nelda Emswiler, RDH
1990

Treat all patients as if they were very special friends, no matter what their station in life is. Leave your prejudices at the operatory door. When you enter, you and your patient are not alone. Someone else is also there working through you if you let them. Although clinical skills are a necessity, they are secondary to interpersonal relationships established with other human beings. Your patients will be uplifted and accept your care and attention with much enthusiasm.

Jeane M. Knowles, RDH
1989

I am a people person. I like to look beyond someone's dentition to really see the person behind the teeth. I show my patients that I care about them as people, in addition to caring about their oral health. If you integrate a patient's total well-being into your practice, then you will find this career as rewarding as I do.

Suzanne G. Ross, RDH
1986

During my 17-year tenure in the dental profession, I have observed a great deal of emphasis being placed on how to make patients feel important and that their dental team cares about them. Some suggestions that I found to be helpful include: using the patient's name; jotting notes in the chart about personal events the patient shares; giving a friendly touch, such as a pat on the shoulder; and calling patients after more aggressive dental procedures.

However, the technique I found to be most effective in communicating to patients that they are important and you sincerely care is to make their best interest your top priority. Patients can tell when you are simply going through the motions and this is not as meaningful as genuine concern and heartfelt compassion.

Myra Cassidy, RDH
1982

This poem made me ponder the importance of something that we, as dental hygiene professionals, strive to give and preserve for our patients.

It costs nothing, but it creates much.
It enriches those who receive without
impoverishing those who give.
It happens in a flash, and the memory of it
lasts forever.
None are so rich that they can get along
without it, and none so poor but are
richer for its benefits.
It creates happiness in the home, fosters
goodwill in a business, and is the
countersign of friends.
It is rest to the weary, daylight to the
discouraged, sunshine to the sad, and
nature's best antidote for trouble.
Yet it cannot be begged, bought, borrowed,
or stolen, for it is something that is not
an earthly good to anyone until it is given
away.
And if in the course of the day, some of your
friends should be too tired to give you a
smile, why don't you give them one of
yours? –Anonymous

Judith A. McCauley, RDH
1973

Don't criticize your patient's home care. It's hard to undo the effects of negative comments. You will make more strides by first acknowledging, in a positive, polite way, that you know they have heard it before. Then express your desire to review home care with them once more in order to ensure that all their efforts aren't in vain.

Pamela Jensen Young, RDH
1988

Be on top of any changes in the laws in your state regarding the profession. Request a new copy of the state regulations periodically. Bring any changes or additions to the attention of your boss and coworkers. They will appreciate being updated as well. Also keep your eyes open as to who has been penalized and for what reason, so that you can address those types of issues in your work environment.

Jane Weiner, RDH
1964

Consider what is in the best interest of your patients at all times. Don't depend on insurance to cover all costs. Provide your patients with all the treatment options and help them choose the best course of treatment.

Tasha Koller, RDH
1999

Always practice good ethics in everything you do, whether it is patient care, infection control, or following state rules and regulations. That way you can sleep at night.

Dori Welch, RDH
1999

Quality is never an accident; it is always the result of high intention, sincere effort, intelligent direction, and skillful execution. It represents the wise choice of many alternatives.
—Willa A. Foster

Linda Harvey, RDH, MS
1973

Chapter Three

Clinical Finesse

Some ways to encourage a patient to become willingly compliant to essential personal daily oral hygiene care are to:

- share the responsibility of noncompliance and show that you really care;
- provide a clear demonstration and explanation;
- never let a patient feel rushed or putoff;
- encourage questions and answer all concerns carefully and patiently;
- make sure the patient understands the seriousness of the inflammation and what can happen if noncompliant;
- maintain an encouraging and reassuring attitude.

Esther Wilkins, RDH, DMD

All of the verbal skills and education available will not convince your patients that they need to proceed with treatment until they take ownership of their oral health. Education and instilling the value of the needed treatment must go hand in hand. This can be as simple as showing the patient the evidence of disease in his or her own mouth.

Cindy Wampler, RDH, BGS
1976

Make your patients comfortable at all times when they are in your chair. For some, it will most likely be their least favorite place. Your goal should be to change their outlook to a positive and enjoyable one by the end of the visit.

Jolie Davis, RDH
1991

Never assume you know someone's condition because you are the dental hygienist. I always review the health history at every visit, even if it's from the day before.

Olivia Willis, RDH
1998

People can afford what they want. It's our job to help patients want the dental work that they need. Besides encouraging them to put their health first, it's good to have some real-life comparisons that they can relate to. For example, when your patient needs bridgework but wants a new car, try relating the cost of the dental work over a period of time to the life span of a car. Hopefully, he or she will see the value of investing in their oral health.

Peg Lehosit, RDH
1976

Teach, teach, teach ...
Never forget the importance of teaching your patients home care. Clean someone's teeth and they will be clean for a day. Teach someone how to clean their teeth and they will be clean for a lifetime.

Cheryl Redmond, RDH
1988

Become a coach. Teaching and preaching run a fine line. Strive to be a motivational teacher and not a floss-pushing preacher.

Jill Obrochta, RDH, BS
1984

When patients find various excuses for not flossing, I explain to them that flossing is a lot like exercise. It may be difficult at first, but if you do it every day it becomes a habit. Getting into the habit of flossing is the best way to ensure good oral health.

Lisa H. Lillis, RDH
1991

Before placing sealants, loosely serpentine a 6- to 8-inch piece of floss interproximately around the teeth that are to be sealed. Then, if any sealant material should happen to flow over between the occlusal contacts, it can easily be removed after curing with a snap upward, breaking the seal that was created between the teeth involved.

Melissa Knowles, BSH, RDH
2000

Flossing orthodontic patients who still have the arch wire can be challenging and tedious. Here's a tip for making it easier. Tie the floss around the floss threader. This not only keeps the floss threader threaded, it also saves time and demonstrates to patients how easy flossing can be.

Barb Chlada, RDH
1986

Floss around abutment teeth and isolated teeth with white 4-ply acrylic yarn. It is very absorbent and the large size collects the plaque and massages at the same time. It can also be used under implant prostheses and on titanium abutments. Acrylic is preferable to natural yarn because natural fibers may break off and become lodged in the sulcus creating a potential for bacterial retention.

Jeane M. Knowles, RDH
1989

Floss a day keeps the hygienist away!

Gina Damico, RDH, MEd
1986

Using disclosing solution is messy and time consuming, but think of how it benefits the patient. Did you always know exactly what plaque was or where to find it? Patients learn a lot from bright pink teeth. It gives them a challenge, something to strive for on their next visit.

Dawn Vonderau, RDH
1998

Pay attention in school when learning how to sharpen instruments. Your instruments are the most important tools you work with daily. If they are not in good shape, neither are you.

Elise Doty, RDH
1994

Don't be afraid of working in a periodontal practice. Little do most hygienists know that this is the type of practice where you can learn the most. Many periodontists love to teach. This provides you with the opportunity to build your skills and greatly expand your knowledge of oral health.

Lynda Shainbrown Richey, RDH
1982

Don't be afraid to hand your patient a toothbrush if, after examining their mouth, you can't see their teeth for the food debris.

Kathy Moore, RDH
1972

Take the initiative to retake your own Xrays before the dentist tells you to. This shows that you are attentive to the quality of your work and the patient care you provide. Disease or decay cannot be found if your Xrays are not as perfect as they should be.

Pam Stevens, RDH
1994

When taking radiographs on patients who gag easily, try these two tips. First, wet the index finger of your glove, then shake salt on it. Put this on the patient's tongue in the area you are taking the Xray and quickly take the Xray. Second, have the patient lift one leg about 6 inches off the foot of the chair while taking the Xray. These two suggestions can be used together for even better results.

Susan Whittaker, RDH
1966

Chapter Four

Making Wise Choices

Making the right employment decision is important. Therefore, keep these three suggestions in mind when interviewing:

- take a list of questions to your interview and make sure all of them are answered before you leave;
- during your interview, take time to interview the employees to determine if they are happy working there;
- don't take the first job that is offered to you unless you are *positive* it is the one for you.

Cammie L. Davidson, RDH, MEd
1985

Try to have a working interview in an office before making a decision. Any office sounds fine until you actually spend time there. This will give you a better understanding of the job you're getting into and the type of people you'll be working with.

Odalis Peters, RDH
1993

Money is not everything. When making an employment decision consider the following:

- go to lunch with the staff—this gives you time outside the office to get acquainted with prospective coworkers;
- spend some time observing in an office—this helps you determine if such things as the office philosophy, infection control, and scheduling practices match your standards and philosophy;
- happiness isn't measured in dollars and cents.

Angie Flood, RDH
1992

Two must-do items that I have relied upon when interviewing are to (1) ask the dentist or office manager if you could contact the former hygienist, and (2) contact the local dental hygiene association placement person before beginning a job search.

Both of these may sound simple, but will save you a lot of wasted time. Over the years, I have found these to be invaluable in eliminating offices that would not be suitable.

Terri Sue Deal, RDH, MS
1966

Regularly put some of your salary into a retirement account. If your employer does not offer a 401K, then start your own. Put as much money as possible in this plan. It is imperative that you save for your future.

Patricia K. Keller, RDH, BS
1967

If you find that you did not make the right employment decision, talk to your employer. Try to discuss issues or concerns in a positive way. If the situation does not seem like it is going to work out, have another job lined up before you quit. Never leave mad, or at least don't let them know that you are. It pays not to burn all of your bridges because you may have to cross them again.

Angela Oakes, RDH
1993

Continually seek to add to your resumé by taking on extra responsibilities outside the clinical realm. You never know when a change will be necessary or beneficial. For example, being the OSHA coordinator for your office could prepare you for a quality assurance position with an insurance company. Experience and knowledge about dental supplies and ordering could lead to a sales opportunity with a dental supply company. Seek to expand your horizons and you will be prepared!

Pamela Moore, RDH
1969

If you can afford to work four days a week, do so. This leaves one day available to substitute in other offices. Doing so provides you the opportunity to network with colleagues in various offices; while broadening your horizon and your skills. If you choose not to work, then you have an extra day to re-energize yourself.

Victoria Barnett, RDH
1981

In all the years I have been practicing hygiene, I have found a gem that continues to be a win-win for the patient, employer, and myself. Although the notion is not a new one, it is one that has motivated me to learn, to grow, and to push myself to stay excited every day. The idea is working with an incentive-based salary. I admit I was not crazy about it at first, but it has proven to be a great idea for everyone, time and again.

I am the a manager of my own "practice within a practice," creating my own destiny. I honestly feel ownership in the practice.

Patty Jordan, RDH
1982

For job security purposes, consider whom you choose as an employer. In my opinion, working for a younger dentist or one who has a family will most likely provide you with long-term employment. As your employer is planning for the future of his or her family, it will most likely provide you security knowing that you can plan for your future as well.

Pam Stevens, RDH
1994

Chapter Five

Professional Partners

Being a good team member is not based on who you know rather it is the result of how you treat those you know.

Tina Daniels, RDH, BS
1971

Over years of working in many different dental offices, I have realized that true job satisfaction can only be achieved in an office where the dentist and his or her employees work together as a team. The contributions that all team members make to the overall success of the practice must be recognized and valued. To attain a sense of pride and accomplishment, all team members must strive toward the common goals of providing excellent dentistry and achieving high standards of patient care.

Kim Kernohan, RDH, BS
1976

I am lucky to work in an office where we all pitch in to help one another, whether it be scrubbing instruments or filing charts. It is important to be a team player because it builds a sense of trust and respect among coworkers and it makes the day go by much smoother. Patients know this and even comment on how much fun we have at work!

Lisa Cerda, RDH
1984

Try to put yourself in the shoes of others. Your coworkers and clients may be having difficulties that you know nothing about that affect their oral health and general disposition. Get them to open up to you as a caring and compassionate professional and friend. They will feel better and you will have a deeper understanding of the fact that you are in this together. You never know when you may need their compassion and understanding.

Katherine Woods, RDH, MPH
1971

Remember to be a team player and not allow yourself to be labeled a prima donna. By focusing on mutual goals you'll get more accomplished for the betterment of the patients and the office. For example, try to learn about various aspects of the office so you can help out when needed and be a true team member.

Bunny Cooney, RDH
1984

Teamwork is an important quality in an office; *always* help one another out. Teamwork encourages improvement in everyone. There is a lot to learn after you graduate. The experience has just begun.

Tasha Koller, RDH
1999

Appreciate your coworkers. Look beyond their weaknesses. Each person in your office has different talents and strengths. Understanding and working with each person's unique behavioral style and personality will help you to grow as a person and, most importantly, to work harmoniously and effectively with other members of your dental team.

Linda M. Harvey, RDH, MS
1973

Service is utmost in a dental practice. It is especially important to those you work with. Serve one another, as you would like to be served. Having an attitude of service indicates that you are part of a whole unit. It includes a willingness to lend a hand when needed, regardless of whose job it is.

Becky Heilman, RDH
1973

Always be a team player ... no one should stand alone.

Jane Weiner, RDH
1964

Chapter Six

Lifelong Learning

Because life is a dance of change we must continually reflect on our faith and beliefs, look for opportunities in every challenge, build enduring relationships, and live to learn continually and to love abundantly.

Gail S. Mitchell, RDH, MPH
1980

Try this: Draw three rows of three dots. Next, try to connect all the dots using only four lines. Can you do it? Here's a hint: you need to go beyond the square to solve it.

Do you ever reflect on what would transpire if you ventured outside your comfort zone? As you mature, are you sticking to what is most comfortable for you, or do you live on the edge ready for change? Are you willing to be open to possibilities that seem a bit different than your beliefs?

As dental professionals, what are your thoughts and, more importantly, actions regarding paradigms learned from experience? Every day you are faced with choices. How do you feel about choosing new products or working with advanced technology?

Realize that the freedom to choose is just around the corner. Are you ready to make the change or is being "in the box" more comfortable? Change is sometimes a challenge. Accept the challenge to explore endless possibilities.

Juli Kagan, RDH, BS
1981

We will continually experience changes in the way we work and play, and in the manner in which we perceive the world. As these changes become more and more dramatic, our roots must remain strong, our mission clearly defined, and our goals and priorities distinct.

Irene Stravos, RDH
1984

As practicing hygienists, it is important that we practice with the best information available. Practicing means we are open to changes and that we are willing for our tomorrows to bring new practices.

Mary Anne Eldreth, RDH, BS
1971

Dental hygiene is a career that is always changing, with numerous opportunities to continue learning. There is variety in clinical dental hygiene, if you seek it. You can create variety within the tasks you do and the little thoughts you say to yourself all day long.

For example, each patient is unique. Discover his or her uniqueness. Remain positive and understanding; don't scold or use guilt to try to change a patient's behavior. Never turn down an opportunity to teach a third-grade class about oral health or to work in a health fair. You meet so many interesting people who may not go to a dentist's office.

Some hygienists change careers because of lack of variety or boredom in daily tasks. Don't let that attitude get a foothold! Ninety-eight percent of the population has gingivitis, how can you be bored? We have so much to offer that can truly make a difference in the health of everyone we touch.

Hazel B. Kerr, RDH, MS
1966

Expand your world! Life is a buffet with many choices so do not be afraid to try new dishes. Develop an appetite for the unique and unusual. When you choose ideas, activities, and suggestions that are not within your usual repertoire, life becomes more than just one repeating day after another.

Helen Douglas, RDH, BS
1978

Do not have tunnel vision. You must be ready to look at new ideas. Some you will use and they will make your job easier or your profession stronger. Some will not be good for your patients or your profession. Learn to tell the difference.

Cheryl Haggerty, RDH
1975

Read dental hygiene journals and keep up with continuing education courses. Patients are very informed consumers these days and hygienists need to keep up with their education.

Susan Follmer, RDH
1966

Remember the importance of lifelong learning. Courses and seminars in dental subjects keep you abreast of new theories and applications, that can be helpful in the practice of dental hygiene. A bachelor's or master's degree can expand your horizons mentally and give you more career options.

Cheryl Masters, RDH, BS
1972

"Knowledge that is not shared is lost."
—Confucius

In our profession, we must be mindful of the fact that we have valuable information to share with our patients every day. Helping others help themselves is a very rewarding part of dental hygiene. As a caregiver, it is also a good idea to take care of yourself by getting involved in an activity, such as yoga, to keep your mind and body healthy.

Donna Yanus, RDH
1985

Take advantage of every opportunity to learn all you can about every aspect of dentistry ... from filing insurance claims to assisting with root canals. The more a hygienist knows, the more valuable he or she is to the practice.

Sheri Miller, RDH
1988

Five years after graduating from dental hygiene school, I obtained a nursing degree. It has really enhanced my dental hygiene career. I feel that I have a greater insight regarding a patient's overall health status, which enables me to provide a higher level of oral health care.

Patricia Baughman, RDH, RN
1990

Commit yourself to lifelong learning. Read professional journals, attend meetings and seminars, take an interest in civic affairs, and become involved. You will find that this widens your circle of influence. Continue learning by becoming an expert in one area of dentistry. It doesn't matter whether it is root planing, data processing, or infection control. Be the person the rest of the staff turns to with questions.

Carroll D. Cameron, RDH, EdD
1960

I have learned through many hours of continuing education that providing more complete services for the patient benefits everyone, including myself. I feel that I have never lost enthusiasm for dentistry because I am constantly learning new ways to deliver better patient care.
As you are inspired to deliver the highest quality of patient care, and as others in the office are additionally energized and involved in this process of care, it truly creates an atmosphere of success for everyone.

Patty Jordan, RDH
1982

There is so much more to oral health and prevention than what we learned in school. What I have discovered is that we need to be assertive, informed regarding the latest research and newest products, and open to change. Recommending a long-term, effective oral hygiene system for our patients to follow at home is the most important part of our job. Don't allow your patients to leave your office only to go to the local drug store and be sold products that they know nothing about, or that contain harmful ingredients.

Our primary job is to educate, and we can only do this if we educate ourselves. I invite all hygienists to join me on this mission!

Michelle Watts, RDH
1977

Chapter Seven

One Last Word

Carpal Tunnel Syndrome and Thoracic Outlet Syndrome are two very real threats to the profession of dental hygiene. Posture and exercise are two important preventive strategies. Beginning each clinical day with simple hand and arm stretches, as well as keeping the best posture attainable throughout the day, will increase chances of warding off these two powerful, adversarial threats.

Holly Hanson, RDH, MS
1976

"Do it now, you become successful the moment you start moving toward a worthwhile goal." —Anonymous

Tracy Weaver, BSDH
1991

Maintain your license even during times you aren't working. You never know when you will decide to return to the profession of dental hygiene.

Swann Knowles, RDH
1938
(first hygienist to serve on the Florida Board of Dentistry)

Never allow another person to make you feel any less than you are, for they are human too.

Jackie Burt McDonough, RDH
1979

Being a member of your professional organization is your lifeline to the heart and soul of the dental hygiene profession.

Tina Daniels, RDH, BS
1971

Always interact with your peers!

"I know of nothing more effective for maintaining a pure heart and keeping one's life balanced and on target than being a part of an accountability group."
—Charles R. Swindoll

"As iron sharpens iron, so one man sharpens another."
—Proverbs 27:17

Codi Kimball, RDH
1975

If I could wish any wish in the world for my beloved profession of dental hygiene it would be that every dental hygienist could know all there is to know about our profession both technically and clinically; could and would serve every patient to the best of their ability as though they were caring for themselves or family; would regard their profession with an attitude of specialty and a willingness to encourage and perpetuate its growth.

That's a big wish, isn't it? Well, after being a full-time hygienist for over half of my life I feel bold, yet humble; to let these strong feelings come out and make themselves quite evident.

As a past president of the Florida Dental Hygiene Association, my theme was "The Hand of Dental Hygiene: The Hand of Empowerment, Friendship and Healing." My chief goal as I traveled around Florida was to inform and challenge dental hygienists to care for our profession, to carry on for our profession, and to join other hygienists to make a difference that would count; thus the "hand of empowerment."

Having graduated from Pensacola Junior College School of Dental Hygiene in 1969 (when it was one of three schools in Florida) was the beginning of my network of friends and colleagues from coast to coast. How wonderful to be able to call a friend/dental hygienist in all parts of the country to compare notes about how particular services or systems are delivered or set up. Sharing ideas and experiences can be a good thing; thus the "hand of friendship."

Giving of oneself to take care of another human being is a bountiful gift one can receive from life. To engage eyes, to give a smile, to approach, to welcome, to give a handshake, to converse, to touch, to make comfortable, to listen, to educate, to show, to instruct, to help learn, to laugh, to enjoy, to encourage, and to praise are just a few of the ways my gift is given. The return on the investment of oneself into this venture of life, I can assure you, is more than any money can buy or any employer can pay you; thus the "hand of healing."

May your personal and professional lives inter-twine and weave such a magnificent cloak that you will always be wrapped with warmth and comfort knowing that you gave your all and did your best.

Susan Halil, RDH
1969

Biography

As a professional consultant and career development coach, Linda Harvey, RDH, MS has devoted her career to helping dental professionals fulfill their goals. Her career as a dental hygienist began in 1973 when she graduated from the State University of New York at Farmingdale. She earned a master's degree in health administration and is licensed as a Healthcare Risk Manager. Linda is the founder and president of Horizon Consulting Group, Inc. She is nationally recognized for her enlightening articles and home study courses and educational programs. Linda is a member of numerous organizations including the American Dental Hygienists' Association, First Coast Healthcare Executives, Toastmasters International, North Florida Professional Speakers Association and the National Speakers Association. Linda dedicates this book to practicing dental hygienists and future hygienists to help them fulfill their personal and professional goals.

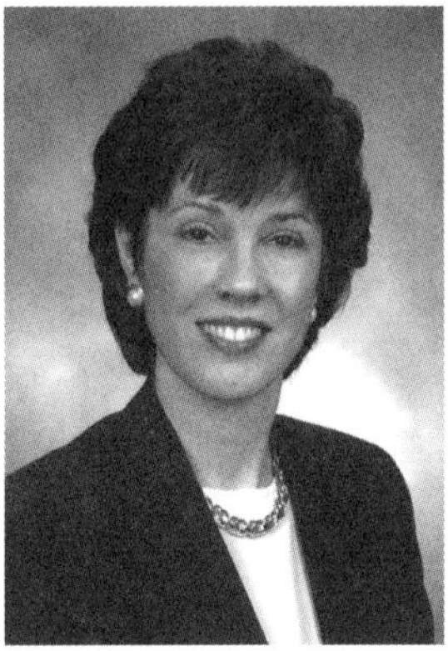

Order Information

Ship to:

Name: ____

Address: ______________________________________

City: ________________ State: __________ Zip: _______

Phone: (____) _________________________________

Email: ____

Please send the following:

Number of book copies ___________________

$12.95 U.S.A. / $19.50 Canadian

Subtotal ___________________

Tax ___________________

(Florida residents only, add 6% sales tax)

Shipping ___________________

(Add $2.50 shipping for the first book, $1.50 for each additional book)

Total ___________________

Send check or money order made payable to:

Horizon Consulting Group, Inc.
Post Office Box 7238
Jacksonville, FL 32238

For availability of speaking engagements or fundraising projects, contact Linda Harvey at Phone/Fax (904) 573-2232 or E-mail: harvey@mediaone.net